I0703254

Energetics of Beauty: Embracing Your Radiant Essence

A Short Guide to Unlocking Your Inner Glow

Halli Star

2024

Table of Contents

Foreword

As a mother of two and a single mom, my journey has been a profound exploration of inner and outer beauty. Living in Mount Shasta, a place that resonates deeply with spiritual energy, I found myself drawn into a transformative experience that awakened me to my true essence.

Mount Shasta became more than just a geographical location; it was a catalyst for my spiritual awakening. In the quiet solitude of its majestic presence, I began to peel back the layers that had obscured my true self. It was here, surrounded by nature's raw beauty, that I started to reconnect with the light within me. This journey wasn't just about finding peace or clarity—it was about rediscovering who I am at the deepest level.

Understanding Our True Nature

When we realize that we are fundamentally made of light, both literally and spiritually, we begin to see that our true beauty comes from within. Our essence is divine, an expression of pure love and light. This understanding encouraged me to value my inner qualities and recognize the deep beauty that resides in my spirit.

Gratitude for the Physical Experience

Our bodies, though temporary vessels, allow us to experience the world in incredible ways. By appreciating the sensations of sight, sound, taste, touch, and smell, we cultivate a mindset of gratitude. This appreciation enhances our inner beauty, making us more mindful and present in our daily lives.

Caring for the Physical Body

Viewing our bodies as sacred temples means treating them with the utmost care and respect. When we nurture ourselves through healthy habits, self-care, and mindfulness, we reflect our inner beauty. A well-cared-for body shines with the light of our inner spirit, showing the world the harmony between our physical and spiritual selves.

Our Mind as a Tool, Not Identity

Our mind is a powerful tool for navigating the world, but it does not define who we are. By releasing negative thoughts and self-doubt, we achieve mental clarity and peace. This inner tranquility is a cornerstone of inner beauty, revealing a calm and centered presence that radiates outward.

Purpose of Life

Embracing love, service, and the remembrance of our true nature aligns us with our inner beauty. Acts of kindness, serving others, and reconnecting with our essence bring out the best in us. These actions reveal the depth of our spirit, showcasing the beauty of our soul in every interaction.

Rediscovery and Growth

Life is a journey of rediscovering our true nature and embracing the experiences that help us grow. This growth is a vital aspect of our inner beauty, characterized by wisdom, compassion, and an enlightened perspective. Each step we take towards self-discovery enhances the radiant essence that defines our true self.

In my journey, I have come to understand human identity formation and spiritual awakening in a deeper context. Initially, we are seen as blank slates, building our identities through experiences within our family, social circles, and education. These experiences shape our perceptions and often lead us away from our true selves. Most people, especially those in their 30s and 40s, go through life identifying with their biographies and personal stories, influenced by external factors and social conditioning.

True awakening involves realizing oneself as a being of light and transcending ego-based emotions and linear time perceptions. This awakening leads to a broader awareness of one's place in the multiverse, not just within their immediate surroundings. Prayer and meditation have been crucial tools for my spiritual growth. Meditation, in particular, has quieted my mind, reduced stress, and brought me closer to my true light body.

Clarity Around the Light Body

As you begin to identify yourself as a being of light rather than just a physical or mental-emotional being, you achieve a deeper awareness of living in the truth. This clarity starts as a thought or concept and evolves into a profound awareness, making your light body brighter. With more light comes more awareness, creating a perpetuating cycle of enlightenment. The more awareness you have, the more light you generate, and this light further enhances your awareness.

Individual awakenings impact the global consciousness. Intuition is vital, and it's important not to identify solely with one's mind and experiences. Substances like sugar and marijuana can hinder spiritual awakening due to their negative vibrational impacts and the attachment of parasitic entities. Embracing a higher spiritual awareness and unity consciousness has been key in my transformation.

Becoming aware of my spiritual essence allowed me to embrace my role as a mother with newfound strength and clarity. I learned to cherish every moment with my children, seeing them as reflections of the divine light that resides within all of us. My journey as a single mom took on a deeper meaning as I navigated life's challenges with a renewed sense of purpose and inner peace.

Through this process, I've come to understand that true beauty emanates from within. It's not just about physical appearance, but about the radiance that shines forth when we connect with our authentic selves. My experiences in Mount Shasta have taught me that embracing our radiant essence is a transformative journey—one that leads to greater self-love, compassion for others, and a profound connection to the world around us.

I invite you to embark on your own journey of self-discovery and inner beauty. May this book serve as a guide and inspiration as you awaken to the light that shines within you.

With love and light,
Halli Star

Chapter 1 The Power Within

Beauty is not just a surface-level phenomenon—it begins deep within you, where your thoughts, emotions, and intentions create a unique energetic signature. In this chapter, we delve into the profound connection between inner energy and outer radiance.

Understanding Your Energy

Your energy is a dynamic force that flows through every aspect of your being. It influences how you feel, think, and interact with the world around you. By becoming aware of your energy, you can harness its power to enhance your natural beauty from within.

Your energy is more than just a physical presence—it's a dynamic force that permeates every aspect of your being, shaping your thoughts, emotions, and interactions with the world. Imagine it as a subtle yet powerful current that flows through you, affecting not only your internal state but also how you resonate with others and the environment.

The Subtle Energy Body

According to ancient traditions and modern holistic practices, humans possess a subtle energy body that interacts with the physical body. This energy body consists of various energetic centers, often referred to as chakras, and meridians that channel energy throughout your system. These energies contribute to your overall well-being, including your mental clarity, emotional balance, and physical health.

Influence on Emotions and Thoughts

Your energy profoundly influences your emotional state and thought patterns. Positive energy fosters feelings of joy, love, and peace, while negative energy can manifest as stress, anxiety, or sadness. These emotional states are not just fleeting experiences but contribute to your overall energy signature, affecting how you perceive yourself and others.

Interacting with the World

Your energy field extends beyond your physical body, interacting with the energies of people, places, and situations around you. Have you ever walked into a room and immediately sensed the atmosphere? This intuitive awareness is often your energy field interacting with the energies present, influencing how you feel and behave in different environments.

Exercise: Tuning into Your Energy

To deepen your understanding of your energy and its influence on your natural beauty, try this simple exercise:

1. **Find a Quiet Space:** Sit comfortably in a quiet room where you won't be disturbed.
2. **Close Your Eyes:** Take a few deep breaths to relax your body and mind. Allow yourself to settle into a calm and centered state.
3. **Scan Your Body:** Begin by focusing your attention inward. Visualize or sense the energy within your body. Notice any areas that feel tense, relaxed, or vibrant.
4. **Notice Your Thoughts and Emotions:** Without judgment, observe your thoughts and emotions as they arise. Notice if they carry a particular energy—positive, negative, or neutral. Allow these thoughts and emotions to simply be, acknowledging their presence without attaching to them.
5. **Expand Your Awareness:** Gradually expand your awareness beyond your physical body. Sense the energy field that surrounds you.

Notice its quality—whether it feels light, heavy, expansive, or contracted.

6. **Set an Intention:** Silently or aloud, set an intention to align your energy with beauty and positivity. Visualize your energy field glowing with a radiant light, symbolizing your inner beauty and vitality.
7. **Reflect:** Take a few moments to reflect on your experience. How did tuning into your energy impact your sense of well-being and inner beauty? Notice any shifts in your mood or perception.

Practicing this exercise regularly can deepen your connection to your energy and enhance your awareness of how it influences your natural beauty. By harnessing the power of your energy, you empower yourself to radiate beauty from within, creating a harmonious balance between your inner essence and outer appearance.

Vibrational Frequency

Every thought and emotion emits a specific vibrational frequency. Positive thoughts and emotions such as love, gratitude, and joy resonate at higher frequencies, radiating outward and enhancing your aura of beauty. Conversely, negative thoughts and emotions can lower your vibrational frequency and dull your glow.

Exercise: Raise Your Vibrational Frequency

1. **Set Up Your Space:** Find a quiet and comfortable space where you can sit or lie down without distractions. You may want to dim the lights and play soft music if it helps you relax.
2. **Center Yourself:** Close your eyes and take several deep breaths. Inhale deeply through your nose, hold for a moment, and exhale slowly through your mouth. Feel yourself becoming more relaxed with each breath.
3. **Focus on Positive Feelings:** Begin by recalling a moment of deep gratitude. It could be a person, a place, or an experience that fills your heart with appreciation. Visualize this memory vividly and feel the warmth and joy it brings.
4. **Expand to Love:** Shift your focus to feelings of love. Think about someone or something you deeply love and cherish. Allow yourself to immerse in these feelings of love, noticing how they radiate from your heart.
5. **Embrace Joy:** Now, think of a joyful moment in your life. It could be a simple pleasure, a funny memory, or a moment of pure happiness. Recall the details of this experience and let the joy bubble up within you.

6. **Visualize Radiance:** Imagine a bright, radiant light at the center of your being, representing your elevated vibrational frequency. Visualize this light expanding outward, surrounding you in a vibrant aura of beauty and positivity.
7. **Release Negativity:** Reflect on any lingering negative thoughts or emotions that may be weighing you down. Acknowledge them without judgment, and consciously release them. Visualize them dissipating into the light, leaving you feeling lighter and more uplifted.
8. **Affirmations of Positivity:** Repeat affirmations that resonate with you, such as "I am love," "I am grateful," or "I radiate joy." Feel the truth of these statements resonating within you, reinforcing your elevated vibrational state.
9. **Gratitude and Closing:** Take a moment to express gratitude for this experience and for the positive energy you've cultivated. Slowly bring your awareness back to the present moment, feeling refreshed and energized.
10. **Integration:** Carry this elevated vibrational frequency with you throughout your day. Notice how it enhances your interactions, perceptions, and inner sense of beauty. Practice this exercise regularly to strengthen your ability to raise and maintain your vibrational frequency.

By regularly engaging in exercises that raise your vibrational frequency, such as this one, you can cultivate a deeper connection to positive emotions and enhance your aura of beauty from within.

Cultivating Positive Energy

To enhance your beauty energetically, cultivate practices that uplift and empower you. This may include mindfulness meditation, affirmations, gratitude exercises, and surrounding yourself with positive influences. These practices not only nourish your soul but also amplify your inner radiance, making you more vibrant and attractive.

Mirror Exercise: Embracing Your Inner Beauty

Find a quiet space where you can comfortably stand in front of a mirror. Take a few moments to center yourself and relax, allowing any tension to melt away.

1. Setting Your Intention

Stand tall and look into your own eyes in the mirror. Set a positive intention for this exercise: to see and appreciate your inner beauty reflected back to you.

2. Deep Breathing

Begin with a few deep breaths. Inhale deeply through your nose, feeling the breath fill your lungs, and exhale slowly through your mouth, releasing any stress or negativity.

3. Affirmations of Self-Love

Repeat affirmations that affirm your beauty and worthiness. Choose affirmations that resonate with you, such as:

- *"I am beautiful inside and out."*
- *"I radiate confidence and grace."*
- *"I am worthy of love and respect."*

Say these affirmations aloud with conviction, allowing their positive energy to permeate your mind and heart.

4. Observation without Judgment

Gaze at yourself in the mirror with a gentle and compassionate attitude. Observe your reflection without judgment or criticism. Notice the unique features that make you who you are.

5. Gratitude and Appreciation

Reflect on three qualities or aspects of yourself that you are grateful for. It could be your kindness, resilience, creativity, or any other positive attribute. Express gratitude for these qualities, recognizing their importance in shaping who you are.

6. Sending Love to Yourself

Visualize sending love and compassion to the person you see in the mirror—yourself. Imagine a warm, golden light surrounding you, filling you with feelings of love, acceptance, and appreciation.

7. Embracing Your Authenticity

Acknowledge and embrace your authentic self. Celebrate your uniqueness and the journey that has shaped you into the person you are today. Allow a sense of pride and self-acceptance to wash over you.

8. Inner Dialogue of Kindness

Engage in a dialogue with yourself, speaking kindly and compassionately. Offer words of encouragement and support, just as you would to a dear friend. Replace any self-criticism with affirmations of self-love and acceptance.

9. Closing Reflection

Take a moment to reflect on how you feel after completing this exercise. Notice any shifts in your perception of yourself and your inner beauty. Embrace the positive energy you have cultivated and carry it with you throughout your day.

10. Integration

Incorporate this mirror exercise into your regular self-care routine. Practice it regularly to strengthen your self-love and appreciation for your inner beauty. Use the mirror as a tool to connect deeply with yourself and affirm your worthiness of love and respect.

Intentional Living

Setting intentions is a powerful way to direct your energy towards specific goals, including enhancing your beauty. By setting intentions for self-love, self-care, and embracing your unique beauty, you align your energy with your desires, manifesting a more radiant and confident presence.

Holistic Approach

 Recognizing that beauty is holistic—encompassing mind, body, and spirit—allows you to approach beauty rituals from a place of authenticity and alignment with your inner self. This holistic perspective encourages practices that honor your whole being, fostering a deep connection between your inner energy and outer appearance.

By exploring and nurturing your inner energy, you lay the foundation for a beauty journey that is not only transformative but also deeply fulfilling. Embrace the power within you to radiate beauty from the inside out, starting with understanding and harnessing your unique energetic essence.

Chapter 2 Rituals of Self-Care

Self-care goes beyond pampering—it's a profound practice that nurtures your mind, body, and spirit, ultimately enhancing your energy and outer beauty. In this chapter, we delve into the transformative power of self-care rituals, exploring how they can elevate your well-being and radiance.

Understanding Self-Care Rituals

Self-care rituals are intentional practices that prioritize your physical, emotional, and mental health. They can range from simple daily routines to indulgent treatments, all aimed at nourishing your holistic well-being. These rituals create a sacred space for you to reconnect with yourself and replenish your energy reserves.

Skincare as a Self-Care Ritual

Your skincare routine is more than just cleansing and moisturizing—it's a ritual of self-love. Taking care of your skin not only improves its appearance but also enhances your confidence and self-esteem. Choose products that resonate with your skin's needs and preferences, turning your skincare routine into a luxurious and nurturing experience.

Mindful Practices for Inner Peace

Incorporating mindfulness into your daily life is a powerful self-care ritual. Mindfulness cultivates awareness of the present moment, reducing stress and promoting emotional balance. Practices such as meditation, deep breathing exercises, or yoga help you center yourself, quiet your mind, and rejuvenate your energy.

Exercise: Affirmations for Mindful Makeup Application

Mindful makeup application can be a powerful self-care ritual that enhances your inner peace and outer beauty. Incorporate affirmations into your routine to cultivate a positive mindset and promote a sense of inner calm. Here's how you can integrate affirmations into your makeup routine:

1. **Prepare Your Space:** Set aside a few minutes in a quiet and comfortable environment where you can focus on yourself without distractions. Gather your makeup products and tools, creating a serene space that encourages mindfulness.

2. **Deep Breathing and Centering:** Begin by taking several deep breaths to center yourself. Inhale deeply through your nose, feeling the air fill your lungs, and exhale slowly through your mouth, releasing any tension or stress.
3. **Affirmations of Beauty and Self-Love:** As you start applying your makeup, repeat affirmations that resonate with you. Here are some examples:
    - *"I am beautiful inside and out."*
    - *"I embrace my unique features and celebrate my natural beauty."*
    - *"Applying makeup is a moment of self-care and self-expression."*
    - *"I am confident and radiant."*
4. **Focus on Each Step:** Pay attention to each step of your makeup routine mindfully. Whether you're applying foundation, enhancing your eyes, or adding a touch of color to your lips, engage fully in the process. Notice the textures, colors, and sensations as you apply each product with intention and care.
5. **Gratitude and Appreciation:** Express gratitude for the opportunity to pamper yourself and enhance your natural beauty. Reflect on the positive qualities you appreciate about yourself and your appearance.

6. **Visualize Your Inner Radiance:** Visualize a radiant light glowing from within you as you complete your makeup look. Imagine this light illuminating your features and reflecting your inner beauty outward.
7. **Closing Reflection:** Take a moment to admire your reflection in the mirror. Appreciate the effort and attention you've invested in yourself during this mindful makeup application. Notice how affirmations have positively influenced your mindset and energy.
8. **Carry Positivity Throughout Your Day:** Throughout the day, recall the affirmations and positive feelings cultivated during your makeup routine. Let them guide you in embracing your inner peace, confidence, and beauty.

By integrating affirmations into your makeup routine, you transform a daily task into a meaningful self-care practice. Mindful makeup application becomes a moment to nurture your inner peace, boost your self-esteem, and enhance your outer beauty with positivity and intention.

Nutrition and Wellness

Nourishing your body with wholesome foods is a fundamental aspect of self-care. Pay attention to what you eat, opting for nutrient-rich foods that support your overall health and vitality. Hydrate your body with plenty of water and herbal teas, promoting radiant skin and a clear mind.

Rest and Relaxation

Restorative sleep and relaxation are essential for rejuvenating your energy and enhancing your beauty. Create a bedtime ritual that promotes deep, restful sleep, such as winding down with a calming book, practicing gentle stretches, or enjoying a soothing bath. Prioritize relaxation techniques that soothe your mind and body, reducing tension and promoting a sense of well-being.

Creativity and Expression

Engaging in creative activities is a form of self-care that nurtures your soul. Whether you enjoy painting, writing, gardening, or dancing - even adult coloring books! Creative expression allows you to connect with your inner self and channel positive energy. Embrace activities that bring you joy and fulfillment, fostering a sense of creativity and inner beauty.

Exercise and Movement

Physical activity is another powerful self-care ritual that enhances your energy and outer beauty. Find activities that you enjoy, whether it's yoga, jogging, dancing, or simply taking a walk in nature. Movement not only strengthens your body but also boosts your mood, promoting a radiant and healthy appearance.

Cultivating Rituals of Self-Care

To incorporate self-care rituals into your life, start by identifying activities that resonate with you and align with your needs. Create a daily or weekly routine that includes a variety of self-care practices, ensuring holistic nourishment for your mind, body, and spirit. Consistency is key—commit to prioritizing your well-being and nurturing your inner and outer beauty through intentional self-care rituals.

By exploring and embracing the transformative power of self-care rituals, you empower yourself to cultivate a deeper connection with your inner self and enhance your radiance from within. Each ritual becomes a testament to your commitment to self-love, promoting a harmonious balance of energy and beauty in your life.

Chapter 3 Aligning with Nature

Nature is not just a backdrop to our lives—it offers profound benefits that can enhance our beauty and well-being. In this chapter, we explore the transformative power of natural ingredients in beauty products and how they resonate with our body's energy, promoting balance and radiance.

The Essence of Natural Ingredients

Natural ingredients derived from plants, minerals, and other organic sources have been revered for centuries for their healing and rejuvenating properties. Unlike synthetic compounds, natural ingredients often contain vitamins, antioxidants, and nutrients that nourish the skin and support overall health.

Here is an example of a homemade body scrub that we love:

DIY Coconut Oil Coffee Scrub Recipe:

Ingredients:

- 1/2 cup coconut oil (solid, at room temperature)

- 1/2 cup ground coffee (freshly ground works best)
- Optional: 1-2 tablespoons brown sugar (for added exfoliation)

Instructions:

1. **Prepare the Coconut Oil:** Measure out 1/2 cup of solid coconut oil and place it in a mixing bowl. If your coconut oil is too firm, you can gently warm it in the microwave for a few seconds until it softens slightly.
2. **Add Ground Coffee:** Add 1/2 cup of ground coffee to the coconut oil. The coffee grounds will act as a natural exfoliant, helping to remove dead skin cells and smooth your skin.
3. **Optional: Add Brown Sugar (for extra exfoliation):** If you prefer a scrub with additional exfoliating properties, add 1-2 tablespoons of brown sugar to the mixture. Brown sugar is gentle on the skin and helps to slough away dry, rough patches.
4. **Mix Thoroughly:** Use a spoon or spatula to thoroughly mix the ingredients together until well combined. Ensure that the coffee grounds are evenly distributed throughout the coconut oil.
5. **Store and Use:** Transfer the scrub into a clean, airtight container or jar for storage. Keep it at room temperature or in a cool, dry

place. Use the scrub within a few weeks for best results.

Before using any homemade skincare products, including this coconut oil coffee scrub, it's important to consider the following safety precautions:

- **Patch Test:** *Perform a patch test on a small area of skin before using the scrub on larger areas. This helps ensure that you don't have any allergic reactions or skin sensitivities to the ingredients.*
- **Skin Sensitivity:** *If you have sensitive skin or any existing skin conditions (such as eczema or psoriasis), consult with a dermatologist before using homemade scrubs.*
- **Avoid Eye Area:** *Keep the scrub away from your eyes and mucous membranes. Rinse thoroughly with water if contact occurs.*
- **Storage:** *Store the scrub in a clean, airtight container at room temperature. Use it within a few weeks to ensure freshness and effectiveness.*
- **Discontinue Use:** *Discontinue use if you experience any irritation, redness, or discomfort after applying the scrub. Consult a healthcare professional if symptoms persist.*

- *Take precaution - coconut oil can be slippery so only apply when you are stable and in a slip free environment.*

Benefits for Skin Health

Natural beauty products are celebrated for their ability to address a wide range of skincare concerns while minimizing the risk of irritation and adverse reactions. Ingredients such as aloe vera, shea butter, coconut oil, and green tea extract are known for their moisturizing, soothing, and anti-inflammatory properties. They help to hydrate the skin, reduce redness, and promote a smooth and radiant complexion.

Harmonizing with Your Body's Energy

Our bodies have an innate connection with nature's rhythms and energies. Natural ingredients resonate harmoniously with our body's energy, aligning with its natural processes and promoting balance. This alignment can enhance the skin's vitality, improve its resilience to environmental stressors, and support its natural regeneration and renewal processes.

Promoting Holistic Wellness

Using natural beauty products goes beyond skincare—it embodies a holistic approach to wellness. By choosing products free from harmful chemicals and artificial additives, you prioritize not only the health of your skin but also your overall well-being. Natural ingredients nourish the skin without disrupting its delicate balance, fostering a sense of harmony and vitality from within.

Environmental Consciousness

Embracing natural beauty products is also a choice that supports environmental sustainability. Many natural ingredients are sustainably sourced and biodegradable, reducing the ecological footprint of skincare practices. By aligning with nature, you contribute to preserving the Earth's resources for future generations.

Spend Time Outdoors

Make a habit of spending more time outdoors, connecting with nature and soaking in its rejuvenating energy. Take walks in parks or natural trails, practice yoga or meditation outside, or simply sit in a garden and observe the beauty of plants and flowers. Spending time in nature not only reduces stress but also enhances your overall sense of well-being, which reflects positively on your skin's health.

The Power of Nature's Vortexes and Cultivating Inner Light

In our journey towards embracing our radiant essence, one of the most powerful practices we can adopt is spending time outdoors, connecting with nature, and soaking in its rejuvenating energy. Nature is not just a backdrop for our lives; it is a vital source of energy and inspiration that can profoundly impact our inner and outer beauty.

The Magic of Nature's Vortexes

Nature is filled with energetic vortexes—special places where the earth's energy is particularly strong. These vortexes, found in places like Mount Shasta, Sedona, and other sacred sites around the world, are believed to amplify our own energy, helping us to align with our higher selves and connect more deeply with the natural world. When we spend time in these powerful locations, we can tap into their energy, allowing it to cleanse and rejuvenate us on a deep level.

Cultivating Energy Within

Just as these vortexes in nature are sources of powerful energy, we too have an inner vortex—a center of light and energy within us that we can cultivate and strengthen. By spending time in nature, we can nourish this inner light, enhancing our overall sense of well-being and vitality. This inner cultivation is not only essential for our spiritual growth but also reflects positively on our physical appearance, particularly the health and radiance of our skin.

Practical Ways to Connect with Nature

1. **Walks in Nature**: Take regular walks in parks or natural trails. Allow yourself to be fully present, observing the beauty around you and feeling the earth beneath your feet. These walks can help ground your energy and provide a sense of peace and balance.

2. **Outdoor Yoga and Meditation:** Practicing yoga or meditation outside allows you to merge your energy with

that of nature. The fresh air, natural light, and sounds of nature can enhance your practice, making it more invigorating and deeply restorative.

3. **Garden Time and Grounding:** Spend time in a garden, whether it's your own or a public one. Engage with the plants, flowers, and the earth. Gardening itself can be a meditative practice, connecting you with the cycles of nature and fostering a deeper appreciation for its beauty and bounty. Additionally, grounding—physically connecting with the earth by walking barefoot on grass, soil, or sand—can charge our energetic body. This direct contact with the earth helps to balance our energy, reduce stress, and enhance our vitality. As we ground ourselves, we absorb the earth's electrons, which help to stabilize our bioelectrical systems. This grounding practice charges our energetic body, enabling us to radiate from within.

By making a habit of connecting with nature, you are not only reducing stress but also enhancing your overall well-being. This connection to the natural world helps you to cultivate your inner light, making you feel more vibrant and alive. As you nourish this inner energy, it radiates outward, illuminating your skin and enhancing your natural beauty.

In essence, the practice of spending time outdoors and connecting with nature is a powerful way to tap into the energetics of beauty. It allows us to align with the rhythms of the earth, cultivate our inner light, and embrace our radiant essence fully.

Incorporating Nature into Your Beauty Rituals

To align with nature in your beauty regimen, consider incorporating products that feature natural ingredients. Look for labels that emphasize organic, plant-based, or ethically sourced ingredients. Experiment with botanical oils, herbal extracts, and mineral-rich clays to discover what resonates best with your skin's needs and preferences.

Practical Application and Tips:

- **Read Labels Carefully:** Familiarize yourself with common natural ingredients and their benefits for skin health.
- **Experiment Mindfully:** Start integrating natural products gradually into your skincare routine to observe their effects on your skin.
- **Consult Professionals:** Seek guidance from skincare experts or dermatologists to tailor natural skincare solutions to your specific concerns.
- **Embrace DIY Beauty:** Explore homemade skincare recipes using natural ingredients to personalize your beauty rituals and enhance your connection with nature.

By aligning with nature, you embark on a journey to discover the beauty-enhancing benefits of natural ingredients. Embrace the synergy between your body's energy and the healing powers of nature, nurturing your skin's health and radiance while honoring the planet we call home.

Chapter 4 The Art of Presence

Beauty is not just a physical attribute but a state of being that flourishes in the present moment. Let's explore how cultivating mindfulness and presence can profoundly enhance your awareness and appreciation of your natural beauty.

Understanding Presence

Presence is the practice of being fully engaged and aware in the present moment, without judgment or distraction. It involves a deep connection with yourself, your surroundings, and the experiences unfolding in the here and now. When you embody presence, you invite a sense of calm, clarity, and authenticity into your life.

The Impact of Presence on Inner Beauty

1. **Cultivating Calm and Serenity:** When you practice presence, you become more attuned to the present moment, allowing you to let go of worries about the past or future. This mindfulness reduces stress and anxiety, which are often reflected in our physical appearance. A calm mind leads to relaxed facial expressions and a serene demeanor,

making you appear more radiant and approachable.

2. **Enhancing Emotional Clarity:** Being present allows you to observe your emotions without getting entangled in them. This emotional clarity helps you respond to situations with grace and composure rather than reacting impulsively. The ability to manage emotions positively influences your interactions with others, making you appear more balanced and harmonious.

3. **Fostering Authenticity:** Presence encourages you to be true to yourself, embracing your genuine thoughts and feelings without judgment. This authenticity is magnetic and attractive, as it fosters trust and connection with others. When you are authentic, your confidence shines through, enhancing your inner and outer beauty.

4. **Improving Self-Awareness:** Practicing presence increases your self-awareness, helping you understand your needs, desires, and boundaries. This self-awareness empowers you to take better care of yourself, making choices that nourish your body and mind. When you honor your well-being, it reflects positively in your physical appearance and overall vitality.

5. **Deepening Connections:** Presence enhances your ability to connect deeply with others. By

being fully engaged in conversations and interactions, you show genuine interest and empathy, which strengthens your relationships. The warmth and compassion you radiate when you are truly present make you more attractive and magnetic to those around you.

6. **Radiating Positivity:** Presence allows you to appreciate the beauty in everyday moments, cultivating a sense of gratitude and joy. This positive outlook on life brightens your demeanor and creates an aura of happiness and contentment. People are naturally drawn to those who exude positivity, as it uplifts and inspires them.

7. **Promoting Physical Well-Being:** Stress and negative emotions can take a toll on your physical health, leading to issues such as dull skin, fatigue, and tension. By practicing presence, you reduce the impact of stress on your body, leading to a healthier, more vibrant appearance. Mindfulness practices like deep breathing and meditation improve circulation and promote a natural glow.

Exercise: Presence Meditation for Radiance

To harness the benefits of presence, try this simple meditation exercise:

1. **Find a Quiet Space:** Choose a peaceful environment where you won't be disturbed.
2. **Sit Comfortably:** Sit in a comfortable position with your back straight and hands resting on your lap.
3. **Focus on Your Breath:** Close your eyes and take a few deep breaths, inhaling deeply through your nose and exhaling slowly through your mouth.
4. **Anchor in the Present:** Bring your attention to the present moment. Notice the sensations in your body, the rhythm of your breath, and the sounds around you.
5. **Observe Without Judgment:** As thoughts or emotions arise, observe them without judgment. Acknowledge them and gently bring your focus back to your breath.
6. **Cultivate Gratitude:** After a few minutes, shift your focus to feelings of gratitude. Reflect on something you appreciate about yourself or your life, allowing this positive emotion to fill your heart.

7. **Radiate Inner Light:** Visualize a warm, radiant light emanating from within you. Imagine this light spreading throughout your body, illuminating your skin and creating an aura of beauty and positivity.

8. **Close with Intention:** When you're ready, slowly open your eyes. Take a moment to set an intention for the day, such as *"I will embrace the present moment with grace and gratitude."*

By integrating presence into your daily life, you cultivate an inner beauty that radiates outward, enhancing your natural attractiveness and fostering a deeper sense of connection and well-being.

Benefits of Cultivating Mindfulness

Mindfulness is a powerful tool that fosters presence by training your attention and awareness. By practicing mindfulness techniques such as meditation, deep breathing, or mindful movement, you learn to observe your thoughts and emotions without attachment. This heightened awareness allows you to appreciate the beauty in everyday moments and connect more deeply with yourself and others.

Enhancing Awareness of Natural Beauty

When you approach life with mindfulness and presence, you develop a heightened sensitivity to the beauty that surrounds you. Whether it's the vibrant colors of a sunset, the delicate scent of flowers in bloom, or the warmth of a genuine smile, you learn to savor these experiences with gratitude and awe. This awareness extends to your own natural beauty, allowing you to embrace and celebrate your unique qualities and inner radiance.

Practical Techniques for Cultivating Presence:

1. **Mindful Breathing:** Take a few moments throughout your day to focus on your breath. Notice the sensation of each inhale and exhale, allowing your breath to anchor you in the present moment.
2. **Body Scan Meditation:** Practice a body scan meditation, where you systematically bring awareness to each part of your body. This helps release tension, improve bodily awareness, and cultivate a sense of presence.
3. **Nature Immersion:** Spend time in nature to reconnect with its rhythms and beauty. Observe the sights, sounds, and sensations around you without distraction, allowing nature to inspire and rejuvenate your spirit.

4. **Gratitude Practice:** Cultivate gratitude by reflecting on the blessings and positive aspects of your life. Expressing gratitude enhances your appreciation for both the simple pleasures and profound experiences that contribute to your sense of beauty and well-being.
5. **Mindful Eating:** Practice mindful eating by savoring each bite of food, noticing its flavors, textures, and nourishing qualities. This mindful approach not only enhances your enjoyment of meals but also encourages a deeper connection with your body's needs and natural rhythms.

Integrating Presence into Daily Life

To incorporate presence into your daily routine, start with small steps that resonate with you. Set aside dedicated time for mindfulness practices, integrate moments of presence into everyday activities, and cultivate an attitude of openness and curiosity toward your experiences. Over time, presence becomes a natural way of being that enriches your life and enhances your appreciation of your inherent beauty.

5-Minute Mindfulness Tip: Putting Your Phone Down to Create Positivity

In our fast-paced world, it's easy to get caught up in the constant stream of notifications and distractions from our phones. Taking just five minutes to put your phone down and practice mindfulness can help shift your focus to positivity and bring a sense of ease and balance to your day. Here's a simple five-minute mindfulness exercise:

Step-by-Step Guide:

1. **Find a Quiet Space:** Choose a quiet, comfortable place where you won't be disturbed. Sit down or lie comfortably, ensuring your posture is relaxed but alert.
2. **Set Your Phone Aside:** Place your phone on silent mode or turn it off completely. Put it out of reach to eliminate any temptation to check it. You can set a timer for 5 minutes before you put it out of reach.
3. **Take a Deep Breath:** Close your eyes and take a deep breath in through your nose, allowing your lungs to fill completely. Hold the breath for a moment, then slowly exhale through your mouth. Repeat this deep breathing three times to settle your mind and body.
4. **Focus on Your Breath:** Let your breathing return to a natural rhythm. Focus your

attention on the sensation of your breath as it enters and leaves your nostrils. Notice the rise and fall of your chest or abdomen with each breath.

5. **Anchor in the Present Moment:** Bring your attention to the present moment. Acknowledge any thoughts or worries that come to mind without judgment. Gently guide your focus back to your breath each time your mind wanders.

6. **Cultivate Positivity:** Think of something positive in your life that brings you joy or gratitude. It could be a recent accomplishment, a loved one, a beautiful memory, or simply the comfort of the moment. Allow yourself to fully experience the positive emotion associated with this thought.

7. **Visualize Positivity Spreading:** Imagine the positive feeling spreading throughout your body, creating a warm and comforting sensation. Visualize this positive energy radiating from you, touching all aspects of your life and interactions.

8. **Set an Intention:** As you near the end of the five minutes, set a positive intention for the rest of your day. It could be something simple like "I will approach my tasks with calm and focus" or "I will spread kindness and positivity in my interactions."

9. **Gently Return:** Take one last deep breath, then slowly open your eyes. Take a moment to notice how you feel and carry this sense of mindfulness and positivity with you as you return to your daily activities.

By dedicating just five minutes to this mindfulness practice, you create a moment of calm and positivity in your day. This exercise doesn't make life's stresses disappear, but it helps you shift your focus to the positive aspects of your life, fostering a sense of ease and well-being. Regularly incorporating this practice can enhance your overall outlook and help you generate more positivity in your life.

By exploring the art of presence, you embark on a journey of self-discovery and inner transformation. Embrace the practice of mindfulness and presence to awaken to the beauty that exists within and around you, fostering a deeper connection with your natural radiance and the richness of each present moment.

Chapter 5 Expressing Authenticity

Your unique essence is your greatest beauty asset. Authenticity and self-expression are powerful tools that can amplify your energy, allowing your inner radiance to shine brightly. In this chapter, we will explore how embracing your true self enhances your natural beauty and provide exercises to help you connect with and express your authenticity.

Understanding Authenticity

Authenticity is the quality of being genuine and true to yourself. It involves embracing your unique traits, values, and experiences without trying to conform to external expectations. When you are authentic, you align with your true self, which brings a sense of inner peace and confidence. This inner alignment radiates outward, enhancing your natural beauty.

The Power of Authenticity

1. **Boosts Confidence:** Embracing your true self boosts your confidence. When you accept and celebrate your unique qualities, you naturally exude self-assurance, which is attractive and magnetic.

2. **Fosters Inner Peace:** Authenticity brings a sense of inner peace as you let go of the pressure to be someone you're not. This tranquility reflects in your demeanor, making you appear more relaxed and approachable.
3. **Enhances Relationships:** Being authentic fosters deeper and more meaningful relationships. When you are true to yourself, you attract people who appreciate and resonate with your genuine nature.
4. **Amplifies Energy:** Authenticity aligns your energy with your true essence. This alignment amplifies your inner radiance, making you more vibrant and alive.

Exercises to Embrace and Express Authenticity

1. Self-Reflection Journal

Purpose: To connect with your true self by reflecting on your values, passions, and unique qualities.

Instructions:

- **Materials Needed:** A journal and a pen.
- **Time Required:** 10-15 minutes daily.

Steps:

1. **Daily Reflection:** Each day, set aside 10-15 minutes to write in your journal. Reflect on the following questions:
   - What are my core values?
   - What activities or hobbies bring me joy and fulfillment?
   - What are my unique strengths and qualities?
   - How do I feel when I am being my true self?
2. **Identify Patterns:** After a week, review your journal entries and identify patterns or recurring themes. This will help you gain a deeper understanding of your authentic self.
3. **Set Intentions:** Based on your reflections, set intentions to incorporate more of your authentic qualities into your daily life.

2. Authenticity Affirmations

Purpose: To reinforce positive beliefs about your authentic self and boost your confidence.

Instructions:

- **Materials Needed:** Sticky notes or index cards.

- **Time Required:** 5-10 minutes daily.

Steps:

1. **Create Affirmations:** Write down positive affirmations that resonate with your authentic self. Examples include:
    - *"I am worthy and enough just as I am."*
    - *"My unique qualities are my greatest strengths."*
    - *"I embrace and celebrate my true self."*
2. **Display Affirmations:** Place the affirmations on your mirror, desk, or any other place where you will see them daily.
3. **Daily Practice:** Each day, spend a few minutes reading your affirmations aloud. Feel the positive energy and confidence they bring.

3. Creative Expression

Purpose: To express your authenticity through creative activities that resonate with your true self.

Instructions:

- **Materials Needed:** Art supplies, musical instruments, writing materials, or any other creative tools.
- **Time Required:** 20-30 minutes weekly.

Steps:

1. **Choose a Creative Outlet:** Identify a creative activity that you enjoy, such as painting, writing, dancing, or playing an instrument.
2. **Set Aside Time:** Dedicate 20-30 minutes each week to engage in your chosen creative activity.
3. **Express Freely:** Allow yourself to express freely without judgment or the need for perfection. Focus on the joy and fulfillment the activity brings.

4. Authentic Communication

Purpose: To practice expressing your true thoughts and feelings in your interactions with others.

Instructions:

- **Materials Needed:** None.
- **Time Required:** Ongoing practice.

Steps:

1. **Be Honest:** In your conversations, practice being honest about your thoughts, feelings, and needs. Speak from the heart and avoid hiding behind a façade.
2. **Listen Actively:** Pay attention to how you communicate and listen to others. Authentic

communication involves both expressing
yourself and genuinely listening to others.
3. **Set Boundaries**: Establish healthy
    boundaries that honor your authentic self.
    Learn to say no when necessary and
    prioritize your well-being.

Expressing authenticity is a journey of
self-discovery and self-love. By embracing your
unique essence, you amplify your energy and allow
your inner radiance to shine brightly. The exercises
provided in this chapter are designed to help you
connect with and express your true self, enhancing
your natural beauty from within. Remember, your
authenticity is your greatest beauty
asset—celebrate it and let it illuminate your life and
the lives of those around you.

Chapter 6 Embracing Your Radiant Essence

As you journey through "Energetics of Beauty," remember that true beauty is a reflection of your inner light. Embrace your radiant essence with intention, self-care, and authenticity. Let Culture Diamond Beauty be your guide to unlocking the beauty that resides within you.

Understanding Your Inner Light

Your inner light is the core of who you are—your spirit, your energy, your true essence. It's the part of you that shines brightly when you are aligned with your values, passions, and purpose. Embracing your radiant essence means honoring and nurturing this inner light, allowing it to illuminate your life and the lives of those around you.

Intention

Living with intention means making conscious choices that align with your authentic self and your highest good. When you set intentions, you create a roadmap for your life, guiding your actions and decisions in a way that supports your well-being and growth.

1. **Morning Reflection:** Begin your day with a moment of quiet reflection. Close your eyes and take a few deep breaths, grounding yourself in the present moment.
2. **Identify Your Focus:** Ask yourself what you want to focus on today. It could be a quality you want to embody (e.g., kindness, patience), a goal you want to achieve, or a way you want to feel.
3. **Set Your Intention:** Clearly state your intention for the day. For example, "Today, I choose to approach every situation with kindness," or "I intend to stay focused and productive."
4. **Visualize:** Spend a few moments visualizing yourself living out this intention. Imagine the positive impact it will have on your day.
5. **Carry It With You:** Throughout the day, remind yourself of your intention and let it guide your actions and decisions.

Self-Care: Self-care is the practice of taking care of your physical, emotional, and mental well-being. It involves listening to your needs and prioritizing activities that nourish and rejuvenate you. Self-care is not a luxury; it's a necessity for maintaining your inner radiance.

Exercise: Creating a Self-Care Routine

1. **Identify Your Needs:** Reflect on what areas of your life need more attention and care. Consider your physical health, emotional well-being, mental clarity, and spiritual growth.
2. **Choose Nourishing Activities:** Select activities that support your needs. This could include exercise, meditation, journaling, spending time in nature, or enjoying a hobby.
3. **Schedule Regular Self-Care:** Set aside regular time for self-care in your daily or weekly routine. Treat it as a non-negotiable appointment with yourself.
4. **Practice Mindfulness:** During your self-care activities, practice mindfulness by being fully present and savoring the experience.
5. **Listen to Your Body:** Pay attention to your body's signals and adjust your self-care routine as needed. Self-care is about being responsive to your changing needs.

Authenticity

Authenticity is about being true to yourself, embracing your unique qualities, and expressing your genuine self. When you live authentically, you align your actions and decisions with your true essence, creating a life that reflects your inner light.

1. **Self-Discovery:** Spend time reflecting on your values, passions, and strengths. What makes you unique? What brings you joy and fulfillment?
2. **Express Yourself:** Find ways to express your authentic self in your daily life. This could be through your style, hobbies, communication, or the way you interact with others.
3. **Set Boundaries:** Establish boundaries that honor your authentic self. Learn to say no to things that don't align with your values and yes to what supports your well-being.
4. **Surround Yourself with Support:** Build a support system of people who appreciate and encourage your authenticity. Let go of relationships that require you to be someone you're not.
5. **Celebrate Your Uniqueness:** Regularly acknowledge and celebrate your unique qualities. Practice self-compassion and self-love, recognizing that you are worthy and enough just as you are.

Final Thoughts

As you conclude your journey through "Energetics of Beauty," remember that true beauty is not about conforming to external standards or striving for perfection. It's about embracing your radiant essence with intention, self-care, and authenticity. By nurturing your inner light, you create a life of beauty, balance, and fulfillment.

At Culture Diamond Beauty, we believe that beauty comes from within. Our mission is to empower you to embrace your true self and shine brightly in all that you do. Let us be your guide on this journey, providing you with the tools, inspiration, and support to unlock the beauty that resides within you.

Embrace your radiant essence. Live with intention. Practice self-care. Express your authenticity. Let your inner light shine brightly, illuminating the world with your unique beauty.

Thank you for joining us on this journey. You are beautiful exactly as you are—let your inner light shine brightly by nurturing and caring for yourself!